Measles Resurgence in Florida:

A Comprehensive Guide to Understanding, Preventing, Responding to, Controlling Measles Outbreaks in Homes and Communities and Events so far.

MARIA D. HENSARD

Table of Contents

Table of Contents   2

Introduction   7

Overview of the Measles Outbreak in Florida   8

Importance of Vaccination and Public Health Measures   9

Chapter One: 12

The Rise of Measles in Florida   12

Initial Cases at Manatee Bay Elementary School   12

Response from Health Officials   14

Controversy Surrounding the

Surgeon General's Decision   15

Chapter Two: Understanding Measles 18

History of Measles and Vaccination Efforts   18

Symptoms and Complications of Measles   20

How Measles Spreads and its Contagious Nature   22

Chapter Three: 25

The Role of Public Health Authorities 25

CDC Guidelines for Measles Outbreak Management   25

State vs. Federal Responses to
Measles Outbreaks   30

Challenges Faced by Health Experts
in Containing Measles   32

Chapter Four: 37

The Impact on Communities   37

Effects of Measles Outbreaks on
Schools and Families   37

Public Perception and
Misinformation About Vaccines: 39

Economic and Social Consequences
of Measles Outbreaks   42

Chapter Five: 45

Lessons Learned and Future Directions   **45**

   Lessons from the Florida Measles Outbreak   **45**

   Strategies for Improving Vaccination Rates and Public Health Education   **47**

   Global Implications of Measles Resurgence   **49**

Conclusion   **52**

Appendix   **59**

Glossary of Terms   **65**

Introduction

In current years, the resurgence of preventable diseases has become a growing concern for public health authorities worldwide. Among these diseases, measles once thought to be under control in many parts of the world, has reemerged as a significant threat to communities, highlighting the critical importance of vaccination and robust public health measures. Nowhere is this resurgence more evident than in the state of Florida, where a recent outbreak has raised alarms and prompted urgent action from health officials.

Overview of the Measles Outbreak in Florida

The measles outbreak in Florida serves as a stark reminder of the persistent threat posed by infectious diseases, even in areas with relatively high vaccination rates. It began with a bunch of cases reported at Manatee Bay Elementary School, located in Weston near Fort Lauderdale. Originally, six children were diagnosed with measles, prompting instantaneous response efforts from local health departments and school officials.

Despite efforts to contain the outbreak, the number of cases continued to rise, with two additional cases reported shortly after. The outbreak underscored the highly contagious nature of measles and the challenges associated with controlling its spread, particularly in densely populated areas such as schools. Concerns grew as the outbreak persisted, raising questions about the effectiveness of vaccination efforts and the need for stronger public health interventions.

Importance of Vaccination and Public Health Measures

Vaccination remains the cornerstone of measles prevention, offering individuals and communities protection against this potentially life-threatening disease. The measles, mumps, and rubella (MMR) vaccine, recommended by the Centers for Disease Control and Prevention (CDC), has been instrumental in reducing measles cases and preventing outbreaks. However, declining vaccination rates in certain communities have contributed to the resurgence of measles in recent years.

The Florida measles outbreak highlights the critical role of vaccination in safeguarding public health. High vaccination coverage not only protects vaccinated individuals but also helps establish herd immunity, reducing the likelihood of disease transmission within a population. By ensuring that a significant proportion of the population is immunized, vaccination programs can effectively contain outbreaks and prevent the spread of measles to vulnerable individuals, such as young children and those with compromised immune systems.

In addition to vaccination, robust public health measures are essential for controlling measles outbreaks and minimizing their impact on communities. Prompt identification and isolation of cases, contact tracing, and targeted vaccination campaigns are key components of outbreak response efforts. Collaboration between public health agencies, healthcare providers, and community organizations is critical for coordinating these efforts and reaching at-risk populations.

Chapter One:

The Rise of Measles in Florida

The resurgence of measles in Florida has brought to light the complex interplay between public health policy, vaccination practices, and community response.

Initial Cases at Manatee Bay Elementary School

The first signs of trouble emerged at Manatee Bay Elementary School, nestled in the suburban community of Weston near Fort Lauderdale. In early reports, it was revealed that six children, attending various grades within the school, had been diagnosed with measles. The news sent shockwaves through the community, as parents and school officials grappled with the realization that a preventable disease had breached the sanctity of their educational institution.

The outbreak at Manatee Bay Elementary School underscored the vulnerability of densely populated environments, such as schools, to the spread of infectious diseases like measles. With children spending the majority of their day in close proximity to one another, the potential for transmission was significant, highlighting the importance of vaccination coverage within educational settings.

Response from Health Officials

In response to the outbreak, health officials at both the local and state levels sprang into action, implementing a series of measures aimed at containing the spread of the virus. Contact tracing efforts were initiated to identify individuals who may have been exposed to the infected children, while vaccination clinics were set up to offer MMR (measles, mumps, and rubella) vaccines to those who had not yet been immunized.

Public health advisories were disseminated through various channels, urging parents to remain vigilant for symptoms of measles and to seek medical attention promptly if their children exhibited signs of infection. School administrators worked closely with health departments to implement hygiene protocols and ensure that affected areas were thoroughly sanitized to minimize the risk of further transmission.

Despite these efforts, the number of measles cases continued to climb, prompting growing concern among health officials and the broader community. Questions arose regarding the effectiveness of vaccination campaigns and the need for more stringent measures to stem the tide of the outbreak.

Controversy Surrounding the Surgeon General's Decision

Amid the escalating crisis, controversy erupted surrounding the decision of Florida's Surgeon General, Joseph Ladapo, regarding the management of the outbreak. In a letter addressed to parents of Manatee Bay Elementary School students, Ladapo asserted that the decision to send children back to school rested with individual parents and guardians, rather than mandating isolation measures recommended by federal health agencies.

This departure from established public health guidelines, which advocate for the isolation of unvaccinated individuals exposed to measles to prevent further transmission, drew sharp criticism from medical professionals and public health experts. Dr. Paul Offit, director of the Vaccine Education Center at Children's Hospital of Philadelphia, condemned Ladapo's stance as prioritizing personal freedom over public health, potentially putting children at risk.

The controversy surrounding Ladapo's decision underscored broader debates surrounding individual liberties, vaccine mandates, and the role of government in public health emergencies. While some applauded Ladapo for championing personal choice and parental autonomy, others expressed concern that his actions could undermine efforts to contain the outbreak and protect vulnerable populations.

Chapter Two: Understanding Measles

Measles, a highly contagious viral infection, has been a persistent threat to public health for centuries.

History of Measles and Vaccination Efforts

Measles, caused by the measles virus, has been recognized as a distinct illness for centuries, with historical accounts dating back to ancient times. However, it wasn't until the 20th century that the measles virus was isolated and identified, paving the way for the development of vaccines to prevent infection.

The first measles vaccine, a live attenuated virus vaccine, was introduced in the 1960s, leading to a dramatic decline in measles cases and associated mortality rates. Subsequent advancements in vaccine technology, such as the development of the measles, mumps, and rubella (MMR) vaccine, further improved protection against measles and contributed to efforts to eliminate the disease.

Global vaccination campaigns, supported by organizations such as the World Health Organization (WHO) and UNICEF, have played a crucial role in reducing measles-related morbidity and mortality worldwide. Despite these efforts, challenges remain, including vaccine hesitancy, limited access to healthcare in some regions, and outbreaks fueled by gaps in vaccination coverage.

Symptoms and Complications of Measles

Measles typically begins with a prodromal phase characterized by fever, malaise, cough, coryza (runny nose), and conjunctivitis (red eyes). This is followed by the development of a characteristic rash, which typically spreads from the head and neck to the trunk and extremities over the course of several days.

Complications of measles can range from mild to severe and may include otitis media (ear infection), pneumonia, encephalitis (brain inflammation), and death. Children under the age of five, pregnant women, and individuals with weakened immune systems are at increased risk of experiencing severe complications from measles.

While most individuals recover from measles without long-term sequelae, the disease can have lasting effects on health and wellbeing. Survivors of measles-associated encephalitis may experience neurological deficits, including intellectual disabilities, seizures, and motor impairments, highlighting the importance of prevention through vaccination.

How Measles Spreads and its Contagious Nature

Measles is highly contagious and spreads through respiratory droplets produced when an infected individual coughs or sneezes. The virus can remain airborne for extended periods, allowing it to infect susceptible individuals who come into close contact with contaminated droplets or surfaces.

One of the key factors contributing to measles' contagious nature is its reproductive number (R_0), which represents the average number of secondary cases generated by a single infected individual in a susceptible population. Measles has an exceptionally high R_0, estimated to be between 12 and 18, meaning that one infected person can potentially transmit the virus to a dozen or more susceptible individuals in an unvaccinated population.

The high transmissibility of measles underscores the importance of vaccination in preventing outbreaks and achieving herd immunity. Herd immunity occurs when a significant proportion of the population is immune to a disease, either through vaccination or prior infection, reducing the overall transmission of the virus and protecting vulnerable individuals who cannot be vaccinated.

Vaccination remains the most effective strategy for reducing the burden of measles and protecting individuals and communities from this highly infectious disease. By prioritizing vaccination coverage, promoting public health awareness, and strengthening healthcare systems, we can work towards the ultimate goal of eliminating measles as a public health threat.

Chapter Three:

The Role of Public Health Authorities

Public health authorities play a crucial role in responding to infectious disease outbreaks, including measles.

CDC Guidelines for Measles Outbreak Management

The CDC serves as the leading authority on infectious disease control and prevention in the United States, providing guidance to public health officials at all levels of government. When it comes to managing measles outbreaks, the CDC has developed comprehensive guidelines to help health authorities respond effectively and minimize the impact of the disease on communities.

Key components of the CDC's guidelines for measles outbreak management include:

1. **Case Identification and Reporting:** Prompt identification and reporting of suspected measles cases are essential for initiating outbreak response measures. Healthcare providers are urged to maintain a high index of suspicion for measles, especially in individuals presenting with fever and rash, and to report suspected cases to local health departments for further investigation.

2. **Contact Tracing:** Contact tracing is a critical component of outbreak control, as it allows health authorities to identify and monitor individuals who may have been exposed to the virus. Close contacts of confirmed measles cases, including household members, classmates, and healthcare workers, are typically advised to monitor for symptoms and, if unvaccinated, receive post-exposure prophylaxis or vaccination.

3. **Isolation and Quarantine:** Individuals diagnosed with measles are advised to isolate themselves from others to prevent further transmission of the virus. In cases where outbreaks are widespread, public health authorities may implement quarantine

measures to restrict the movement of exposed individuals and prevent the spread of infection within communities.

4. **Vaccination Campaigns:** Vaccination remains the most effective means of preventing measles outbreaks. The CDC recommends routine vaccination with the measles, mumps, and rubella (MMR) vaccine for all children, with the first dose administered at 12-15 months of age and the second dose at 4-6 years of age. During outbreaks, targeted vaccination campaigns may be conducted to increase immunization coverage among at-risk populations.

5. **Public Communication and Education:** Clear and timely

communication with the public is essential for promoting awareness of measles risks, encouraging vaccination, and providing guidance on preventive measures. Health authorities are encouraged to utilize various communication channels, including social media, press releases, and community outreach efforts, to disseminate accurate information and address concerns.

By adhering to these guidelines, public health authorities can effectively mitigate the impact of measles outbreaks and protect the health and well-being of individuals and communities.

State vs. Federal Responses to Measles Outbreaks

In the United States, the management of infectious disease outbreaks involves collaboration between state and federal health agencies. While the CDC provides overarching guidance and support, state and local health departments are primarily responsible for implementing outbreak response measures and coordinating efforts on the ground.

State responses to measles outbreaks may vary depending on factors such as the severity of the outbreak, local vaccination coverage rates, and available resources. Health authorities may declare public health emergencies, mobilize healthcare providers to administer vaccines, and implement control measures such as school exclusions and quarantine orders to limit the spread of the virus.

At the federal level, agencies such as the CDC and the Department of Health and Human Services (HHS) provide technical assistance, epidemiological support, and funding to support state-led response efforts. Federal agencies may also coordinate multi-state outbreak investigations, deploy rapid response teams to affected areas, and assist with vaccine distribution and procurement.

Despite the collaborative nature of outbreak response efforts, tensions between state and federal authorities may arise, particularly in cases where there are differences in opinion or approach. Conflicting priorities, jurisdictional disputes, and political considerations can complicate coordination and hinder the effectiveness of response efforts.

Challenges Faced by Health Experts in Containing Measles

Containing measles outbreaks presents numerous challenges for health experts, ranging from logistical and operational hurdles to broader societal and political factors. Some of the key challenges include:

1. **Vaccine Hesitancy:** Vaccine hesitancy, fueled by misinformation and mistrust of vaccines, remains a

significant barrier to achieving high immunization coverage rates. Addressing vaccine hesitancy requires targeted communication strategies, community engagement efforts, and partnerships with trusted leaders and influencers.

2. **Resource Constraints:** Limited resources, including funding, personnel, and infrastructure, can constrain the ability of health authorities to mount an effective response to measles outbreaks. Adequate investment in public health infrastructure and preparedness is essential for building resilience and ensuring timely and coordinated responses to emerging threats.

3. **Globalization and Travel:** The interconnected nature of global travel and trade can facilitate the rapid spread of infectious diseases like measles across borders. Health authorities must remain vigilant for imported cases and implement measures such as border health screening and surveillance to prevent the introduction and spread of measles within their jurisdictions.

4. **Health Inequities:** Socioeconomic disparities, access barriers, and structural inequities can exacerbate vulnerability to measles outbreaks among marginalized and underserved populations. Addressing health inequities requires a comprehensive approach that addresses underlying

determinants of health and ensures equitable access to healthcare services and resources.

5. **Misinformation**: The proliferation of misinformation and conspiracy theories about vaccines and infectious diseases can undermine public trust in public health interventions and fuel vaccine hesitancy. Health authorities must counter misinformation with evidence-based messaging, transparent communication, and proactive efforts to engage with communities and address concerns.

In the face of these challenges, health experts must remain vigilant, adaptable, and collaborative in their efforts to contain measles outbreaks and protect public health. By leveraging scientific expertise, data-driven strategies, and community partnerships, health authorities can work together to mitigate the impact of measles and other infectious diseases on individuals and communities.

Chapter Four:

The Impact on Communities

Measles outbreaks have profound effects on communities, extending beyond individual health to encompass social, economic, and educational dimensions.

Effects of Measles Outbreaks on Schools and Families

When measles strikes a community, schools often find themselves at the forefront of the response efforts. The presence of the virus in educational settings raises concerns about the safety of students and staff, prompting school administrators to implement measures to prevent further transmission. These measures may include temporary closures, enhanced hygiene protocols, and vaccination campaigns aimed at increasing immunization coverage among students and staff.

The disruption caused by measles outbreaks can be significant, leading to interruptions in learning, extracurricular activities, and routine school operations. School closures can also place a burden on working parents who must arrange for alternative childcare or take time off from work to care for their children.

For families directly impacted by measles, the experience can be emotionally and financially taxing. Parents may worry about the health and well-being of their children, particularly if they are too young to be vaccinated or have underlying health conditions that put them at greater risk of complications. The need for isolation and medical care further disrupts daily routines and may strain familial relationships. Additionally, families may face financial strain due to medical expenses associated with treating measles cases and the potential loss of income resulting from missed workdays.

Public Perception and Misinformation About Vaccines:

Measles outbreaks often trigger public debates about vaccination, fueling concerns about vaccine safety and efficacy. Misinformation and misconceptions about vaccines can spread rapidly through social media and other online platforms, contributing to vaccine hesitancy and undermining trust in public health authorities.

One of the most persistent myths surrounding vaccines is the debunked link between the MMR vaccine and autism, perpetuated by discredited research and celebrity endorsements. Despite overwhelming scientific evidence refuting this claim, many individuals continue to express skepticism about the safety of vaccines, leading to suboptimal vaccination rates and increased susceptibility to measles outbreaks.

Public perception of vaccines is further influenced by cultural beliefs, religious convictions, and personal experiences with healthcare providers. Addressing vaccine hesitancy requires a multifaceted approach that acknowledges and respects diverse perspectives while providing accurate information about the benefits and risks of vaccination.

Health authorities and community leaders play a crucial role in combating vaccine misinformation and promoting vaccine acceptance. By engaging with communities, addressing concerns, and emphasizing the importance of vaccination for individual and community health, public health officials can help mitigate the impact of measles

outbreaks and prevent future outbreaks
from occurring.

Economic and Social Consequences of Measles Outbreaks

Measles outbreaks can have far-reaching economic and social consequences, affecting not only individuals and families but also businesses, healthcare systems, and broader societal institutions. The direct costs of treating measles cases, including medical expenses and lost productivity, can place a strain on healthcare resources and exacerbate existing healthcare disparities.

Indirect costs associated with measles outbreaks may include reduced consumer spending, decreased tourism revenue, and disruptions to workforce productivity. Businesses may experience declines in sales and profits as consumers avoid public spaces and limit travel due to concerns about contracting measles. Additionally, healthcare providers may face increased demand for services related to measles diagnosis, treatment, and vaccination.

Socially, measles outbreaks can deepen divisions within communities and erode trust in public institutions. Stigmatization of affected individuals and communities may occur, perpetuating fear and discrimination. Moreover, the politicization of vaccine-related issues can polarize public opinion and hinder collaborative efforts to address the underlying causes of vaccine hesitancy.

Addressing the impact of measles outbreaks requires a coordinated and complete strategy that prioritizes vaccination, facilitates accurate information, and fosters community stability. By recognizing the interconnectedness of health, social, and economic factors, communities can work together to mitigate the effects of measles outbreaks and build a healthier, more resilient future.

Chapter Five:

Lessons Learned and Future Directions

The measles outbreak in Florida has served as a sobering wake-up call, prompting reflection on the lessons learned and charting a course for future public health strategies.

Lessons from the Florida Measles Outbreak

The outbreak in Florida has underscored the fragility of our defenses against vaccine-preventable diseases and highlighted areas for improvement in public health preparedness. One of the key takeaways from the outbreak is the importance of early detection and brisk response. Timely identification of cases, coupled with assertive measures such as contact tracing and targeted vaccination campaigns, can help contain outbreaks before they spiral out of control.

Furthermore, the outbreak has demonstrated the critical role of effective communication and collaboration between public health authorities, healthcare providers, and community stakeholders. Precise and evident communication is essential for building trust and ensuring that accurate information reaches the public, particularly in the face of misinformation and vaccine hesitancy.

Another important lesson from the outbreak is the need for continuous monitoring and surveillance of vaccine coverage rates and disease incidence. By closely tracking these metrics, public health officials can identify vulnerable populations and hotspots for disease transmission, allowing for targeted interventions to prevent outbreaks.

Strategies for Improving Vaccination Rates and Public Health Education

In light of the measles outbreak, efforts to improve vaccination rates and public health education must be prioritized. One strategy is to enhance access to vaccines by expanding vaccination clinics, particularly in underserved communities where access to healthcare may be limited. Outreach efforts targeting high-risk populations, such as unvaccinated individuals and those with vaccine hesitancy, can help address disparities in vaccine coverage and improve community immunity.

Furthermore, public health education movements aimed at dispelling myths and misconceptions about vaccines are essential for building trust and confidence in immunization. These movements should leverage evidence-based messaging and engage with society leaders and influencers to effectively communicate the importance of vaccination in safeguarding individual and community health.

Integrating comprehensive vaccine education into school curricula can help instill a lifelong commitment to immunization and foster a culture of health and prevention from an early age. By empowering individuals with accurate information about vaccines and their role in preventing disease, we can combat misinformation and strengthen vaccine acceptance within communities.

Global Implications of Measles Resurgence

The resurgence of measles in Florida is not a solitary occurrence but rather part of a broader global trend. Measles outbreaks have been reported in multiple countries around the world, fueled by elements such as vaccine hesitancy, limited access to healthcare, and gaps in immunization coverage.

The global implication of measles resurgence underscores the interconnectedness of health systems and the need for coordinated international efforts to address vaccine-preventable diseases. Collaboration between countries, sharing of best practices, and support for vaccination programs in low-resource settings are critical for achieving global measles control and elimination goals.

Furthermore, the resurgence of measles highlights the importance of pandemic preparedness and response efforts. The same principles and strategies used to combat measles outbreaks, such as surveillance, vaccination, and public health communication, are applicable to other infectious diseases, including emerging pathogens with pandemic potential.

Conclusion

In conclusion, the measles outbreak in Florida serves as a poignant reminder of the critical importance of vaccination and disease prevention efforts in safeguarding public health. Throughout this exploration of the outbreak and its implications, several key points emerge, underscoring the need for proactive measures and collaborative action to address vaccine-preventable diseases like measles.

Summary of Key Points

Firstly, the outbreak highlighted the contagious nature of measles and the potential for rapid transmission within communities, particularly in settings such as schools where individuals come into close contact with one another. This underscores the importance of vaccination coverage in maintaining herd immunity and preventing outbreaks.

Secondly, the response from public health authorities at both the local and state levels shed light on the challenges faced in containing the spread of measles and the importance of early detection, contact tracing, and targeted vaccination efforts. However, controversies surrounding decision-making processes also highlighted the need for clear communication and alignment with evidence-based guidelines.

Furthermore, the impact of measles outbreaks extends beyond immediate health consequences, with implications for schools, families, and broader societal dynamics. The disruption caused by outbreaks can strain healthcare resources, disrupt educational systems, and exacerbate economic and social inequalities.

Moreover, the outbreak underscored the prevalence of vaccine hesitancy and misinformation, which pose significant barriers to achieving optimal vaccination coverage and herd immunity. Addressing these challenges requires comprehensive public health education campaigns, community engagement efforts, and policies that promote vaccine acceptance and accessibility.

Call to Action for Vaccination and Disease Prevention

In light of these observations, it is imperative that we heed the lessons learned from the Florida measles outbreak and take decisive action to strengthen vaccination efforts and disease prevention strategies. This includes:

1. **Promoting vaccination as a fundamental pillar of public health:** Vaccination remains one of the most effective tools we have in preventing infectious diseases like measles. It is essential that individuals, families, and communities prioritize vaccination as a vital component of maintaining overall health and well-being.

2. **Enhancing public health infrastructure and preparedness:** Investing in robust public health infrastructure, including surveillance systems, vaccination programs, and emergency response mechanisms, is crucial for effectively detecting, responding to, and mitigating the impact of infectious disease outbreaks.

3. **Combatting vaccine hesitancy and misinformation:** Addressing vaccine hesitancy requires a multifaceted approach that includes providing accurate information about vaccines, addressing concerns and misconceptions, and building trust in the healthcare system. Community engagement, dialogue, and

collaboration with trusted sources can help dispel myths and promote vaccine acceptance.

4. **Fostering global cooperation and solidarity:** Infectious diseases like measles do not respect borders, underscoring the importance of international collaboration in combating disease outbreaks. Supporting global vaccination efforts, sharing best practices, and strengthening health systems in low-resource settings are essential for achieving global health security.

In conclusion, the Florida measles outbreak serves as a stark reminder of the ongoing threat posed by vaccine-preventable diseases and the critical importance of vaccination and disease prevention efforts. By working together to address the root causes of vaccine hesitancy, strengthen public health infrastructure, and promote vaccine acceptance, we can build a healthier and more resilient future for all.

Appendix

As we conclude our exploration of the measles outbreak in Florida and its broader significance, here are more resources to deepen your understanding of measles, vaccination, and public health. Below are suggested resources for further reading and information:

1. **Centers for Disease Control and Prevention (CDC):** The CDC's website offers extensive information on measles, including vaccination guidelines, outbreak updates, and resources for healthcare providers and the public. Visit www.cdc.gov/measles for more information.

2. **World Health Organization (WHO):** The WHO provides global data on measles cases, vaccination coverage, and strategies for measles control and elimination. Explore www.who.int/immunization/diseases/measles/en/ for insights into global efforts to combat measles.

3. **American Academy of Pediatrics (AAP):** The AAP offers guidance for healthcare providers and parents on measles vaccination, disease prevention, and outbreak management. Visit www.aap.org/en-us/Pages/Default.aspx for valuable resources.

4. **National Institutes of Health (NIH):** The NIH conducts research on measles, vaccine development, and

public health interventions. Explore www.nih.gov for the latest scientific publications and studies related to measles.

5. **Local Health Departments:** Contact your local health department for information on measles vaccination clinics, outbreak updates, and community resources. Your health department can provide personalized guidance and support based on your location.

6. **Educational Institutions:** Universities and academic institutions often publish research articles, educational materials, and public health initiatives related to measles and vaccination. Explore university

websites and libraries for valuable resources.

7. **Nonprofit Organizations:** Nonprofit organizations dedicated to immunization advocacy and public health education, such as Vaccinate Your Family and the Immunization Action Coalition, offer educational materials, webinars, and toolkits for healthcare professionals and the public.

Timeline of Major Measles Outbreaks:

Below is a timeline of significant measles outbreaks throughout history, illustrating the impact of the disease and the evolution of vaccination efforts:

- **1963-1965:** The introduction of the measles vaccine in the United States leads to a significant decline in measles cases.

- **1989-1991:** A large measles outbreak occurs in the United States, primarily affecting unvaccinated children and resulting in renewed efforts to improve vaccination coverage.

- **2014-2015:** Measles outbreaks linked to Disneyland in California spark national attention and highlight the importance of vaccination in preventing outbreaks.

- **2019**: The World Health Organization declares measles outbreaks a global health crisis, citing significant increases in cases worldwide and highlighting gaps in vaccination coverage.

- **2021-2022:** Measles outbreaks occur in multiple countries, including the United States, highlighting ongoing challenges in measles control and elimination efforts.

Glossary of Terms

To aid in understanding key concepts discussed in this book, below is a glossary of terms related to measles, vaccination, and public health:

1. **Measles**: A highly contagious viral infection characterized by fever, rash, cough, and other symptoms.
2. **Vaccination**: The administration of a vaccine to stimulate the immune system and provide protection against specific diseases.
3. **Herd Immunity:** A form of indirect protection from infectious diseases that occurs when a large percentage of

a population becomes immune, reducing the spread of the disease.

4. Outbreak: The occurrence of cases of a particular disease in excess of what is normally expected within a specific geographic area or population.

5. **Immunization**: The process of becoming immune or resistant to a specific infectious disease through vaccination.

6. **Public Health:** The science and practice of protecting and improving the health of communities through education, promotion of healthy behaviors, and disease prevention.

7. **Epidemiology**: The study of the distribution and determinants of health-related states or events in

populations, and the application of this study to control health problems.